Zero Belly Diet Book

Discover How to Get a Flat Belly Fast

Simple Ways to Lose Weight and Live Healthy

By

WaraWaran Roongruangsri

Pawana Publishing

Good Health Content

Part of the secret of success in life is to eat what you like and let the food fight it out inside.

-Mark Twain

CONTENTS

AUTHOR'S NOTE

Excess belly fat has an effect on your appearance for sure. Moreover, it affects your overall health. So the book 'Zero Belly Diet' is important for you.

The book includes valuable information that you should know about fat belly. It includes tips and advice that will help you to lose fat and drop your fat belly. You will get more information on losing fat belly in each issue of the 'Zero Belly Diet' book.

In this issue of 'Zero Belly Diet' book, you will get to know about the below mentioned topics.

- How important is to eat the right foods so that you can get rid of the fat deposits in your belly
- Effective and easier diet plan to reduce the belly fat
- Motivational tips to stay on your diet and get the desired results in a much simpler way

'Zero Belly Diet' is the book you can't miss as it includes step by step report on maintain a healthier lifestyle. It helps you to understand the natural ways of leading a healthy lifestyle which can be followed by anybody. After all, you need a positive attitude to switch to a better lifestyle. The book will guide you with easier ways that you can follow it without much effort.

Do you mind drinking extra few cups of water daily? Can't you think you can count your calories? What about getting up from your softy couches and taking a walk outside? If you can do simple steps like, then you are already on the path of leading a healthier lifestyle.

Here ends your search for ways to get back in shape. This is a perfect guide that will help you to stay fit and feel good about yourselves. It is easy for anyone to follow the basic steps in this book. It helps you to lose your extra pounds in simpler ways. Not only will you look great, you will feel great too!

Thanks for downloading the book! I am sure you will enjoy it!

Happy Reading!

WaraWaran Roongrungsri

INTRODUCTION

How many times do you see yourself in front of the mirror? Do you feel like looking a little better than you do now? Well, the answer will probably be yes. You are not alone while you think so. There are many people who want to look better through simpler ways.

It is a growing concern that the craving for fatty foods and lack of proper exercise has resulted in the deterioration of our health, particularly when North Americans are considered. In olden days, we used to indulge in physically demanding jobs or heavy labor that would take away the major part of a day. We exhausted ourselves, which in turn helped in burning out the extra calories in our body.

The scenario is different today. Technology has changed our lives immensely and we live a life of less body exertion. We follow a lifestyle that we all enjoy, but may suffer later due to ill health. Kids are often glued to the computer screen with super powered video games or endless social networking groups, which prevents them from playing outdoor games. The upcoming generation is also expected to follow a similar lifestyle which keeps the health of the body at risk.

On the other hand, the weight loss industry is booming by marketing massively bogus ineffective and instant-result causing fat loss products. People often spend huge amounts by falling prey to this numerous marketing techniques. They think they will get the results similar to what they advertise and pour thousands of dollars into the market. Few people realize the fact that there is no instant resulting fat loss products and many of the diet fads does not work at all.

So what works in life? It is definitely a single thing and that is called hard work. But it is certainly not hard as you think when you hear the word. By hard work, it is meant to think positively and take the necessary steps rather than ignoring reality and going behind products of no use.

If you can get incredible results out of a simple diet and a bit of exercise, then it would be far better than going behind such products. The reason for people to quit the diet plan is because they want the result instantly. Nothing would happen immediately and it takes time for the body to burn out the extra calories and make you fit. You need will power to stay on a diet plan. If you have a strong will to lose your pounds and get in shape, you will surely reach your goals.

The following steps will help you to achieve your goals. Stay focused, concentrate on your goals and above all have a positive attitude! It will do wonders on you!

1. HOW MUCH FOOD YOU NEED?

Do you know how much food you consume in a day? Do you realize how much high-calorie or fatty foods you have each day, even without knowing it? Well, try out this simple way to calculate the intake of food daily. Identify the nutrition facts on the packages of food you eat and note down each day. Continue to note it for a week and try to understand the things that have gone wrong in your eating habits. By calculating the intake of food each day, you will get to realize and analyze the ways to improve the diet.

Often we tend to ignore the proper nutritional foods and go behind those delicious foods that tickle our taste buds. Another reason for the attraction towards the fast food is that it far more convenient to get as opposed to spending so much time in the kitchen to make a tasty dish. Ultimately, this will lead to overweight or obesity. The convenience factor is the sole reason behind the increasing cases of obesity, which happens to be an unfortunate reality. That explains the importance of monitoring the food intake. It will help to realize the areas that need attention.

The perfect start for a healthier lifestyle is to start by analysing the quantity of food each day. Slowly, you can start analyzing the nutrition contained in your daily diet and realize the foods that make you obese. You can start to diminish the fat deposits in your body and switch to healthier foods.

Here is a price of information that might help you. A pound of fat approximately equals to 3500 calories. Suppose your target is to lose a pound of fat in one week. Then you have to reduce 500 calories per day for a week by limiting food intake and replacing it with healthier food stuff. Adding to it, you can incorporate physical exercise of 30 to 45 minutes in your routine. On the first day of the new routine, you will be down to 2500 and then you can devote a few minutes for biking, running, or even an elliptical. The next day you will come to 2000 calories by following the healthier meal plan along with cardio-training. After seven days, you will lose 2 lbs from the overall weight of your body. Moreover, you will experience freshness in body as well as mind. By putting a little effort each day, you will reach your goals.

You will head towards a healthier lifestyle by spending few hours in physical exercises. Your entire body, including heart will enjoy a great workout in the process. As said before, limiting food intake, eating healthier food stuffs and engaging in physical exercises will do wonders on your body and mind. It will definitely. You will experience a higher level of self confidence and also, vote of confidence from people around you. In fact, a simple change in routine life will result in the improved quality of life.

On the other hand, if you opt to go on a food strike to get back in shape it may turn disastrous. You will feel hungrier and may turn lethargic at first. You may experience hunger pains too. Over the time, you will get into a serious eating binge.

The result of a lifestyle with healthier foods and doing exercise regularly is guaranteed as it is one of the tried and tested methods to lose weight and stay fit.

2. A HEALTHIER CHOICE!

As a first step, you will discover the unwanted calories you eat every day knowingly or unknowingly. What is next step? Well, the appropriate step is to find out where you have to make adjustments in the diet. It should be evaluated in such a way that healthier food will replace the fats in your diet.

Wondering how to make it practical? Consider a situation when you are offered a McDonald's Big Mac. It constitutes of higher level of calories as well as lots of bad ingredients. It is better to replace it with a hamburger. It is not essentially a healthy food, but much lower in calorie content and healthier when compared to the former.

Let us consider another example of flamed-broiled Whopper at Burger King. It comes bigger in size than the Big Mac and contains 750 calories and 50 grams of fat in a single piece itself. Switch to a mayo free Whopper of smaller size. That will help you to limit 480 calories and 36 grams of fat in a simple meal. By this way you can avoid the larger sized fries and eat a smaller portion, so that your intake of calories became less. Are you doubtful that you may feel hungry again? Then go for an apple or a bowl of grapes or even a second burger.

There are few fast food restaurants which would offer healthier food options for you. A popular example is KFC, where you will get grilled chicken. The grilled chicken breast and drumstick added with mashed potatoes and gravy in KFC approximately constitutes 400 calories and 12 grams of fat. If you would like to opt for crispy chicken breast, which is tastier than the other, includes 500 calories and over 30 grams of fast since it is deep fried.

If you like to have pizza, then go for a thin crust at Domino's. Make sure you spice it up with ham and pineapple and not pepperoni. It will help you to limit almost 200 calories in your food intake.

Do you go behind milk shakes to quench your thirst? Well, it is a delicious drink for anyone. You do not need to avoid a tasty drink like ilk shake if you are on a healthier diet. Instead you can opt for a smaller sized cup. Here is the reason. A king sized cup of triple thick strawberry shake will contain almost 1000 calories while a small sized cup comes with 420 calories. It makes clear that by opting for a smaller sized cup, you are limiting calories. If you want better results, then prefer an orange juice rather than milk shake.

Let us discuss about breakfast now. It is the starting meal which is very essential to energize and prepare you for the demanding schedules of the day. For Americans, egg McMuffin is a popular choice of breakfast. It contains 300 calories while the English muffin includes 150 calories. This is how you can switch to lesser calorie food items and thereby get the desired results.

It does not mean that the above suggested food items are healthier choices. Somehow it will help to reduce the intake of calories by switching to down-sizing the quantity. It will ultimately lead to the weight loss.

The people of America always get fascinated with fast food. It is pretty easy to get while you are on your way to office as opposed to search in fridge for items to cook a healthy meal. The trouble of cooking as well as time can be saved when you opt fast foods. It is all around you, no matter where you are.

Even when you go behind fast foods also, you can find the healthy foods in it. You always have an option to limit intake of those foods by picking up it in small quantities.

Probably, every food that comes to you will have its nutritional values printed on the package. The advantage is you can closely watch the food you eat rather than finding faults in the fast food industry or even blaming other factors that prevent you from losing your weight. Fast food has many advantages in our busy life style. It is completely left to you to monitor the calories, choose the right one, limit the food intake, and thereby switch to a healthier lifestyle.

Shedding pounds is only the start of healthier lifestyle. It is very important to stay in the improved eating habits. You will always have a temptation to have junk foods or snacks in between meals. There is no problem if you eat it in limited quantities while your normal meals are in a healthy manner. It is very normal to feel hungry and there is no point in struggling with the craving for the food. But make sure you exercise regularly and enjoy a reasonably healthy diet, if you are aiming at the proper health of the body and mind.

3. REDUCING YOUR MEALS!

After going through the previous two chapters, you might have got the point that switching to small sized meals definitely has a major role in weight loss. It has been scientifically proven that once you reduce the quantity of food intake, your body will experience a steady metabolic rate. Start on a habit of eating six to seven meals a day rather than two or three meals of high calories.

Do you own a habit of munching the snacks that come in packets, like potato chips? It will be surely in a mega sized pack. Most people enjoy eating it even when your hunger is satisfied. You will have a tendency to eat more than what your body really needs. Unluckily, you will not have the amount of calories you consume while opening up a packet of potato chips in front of you. In order to stop it, always take a small portion out in a bowl before you eat. You can also add some fruit to realize the amount of food you need.

It has to be taken note that most of the food packets come

in super sized packages and not in small size. Even you walk to a restaurant you will see most items are served in super size, which is obviously greater the quantity of what our body needs. Don't you think the rising statistics of obese people are directly proportional to the size of the packages?

Normally, we go behind tasty foods, but we never realize that we are putting our health at risk by doing it. That explains the importance of switching to small sized foods when compared to larger packets. So you will enjoy delicious food, but will be able to get rid of bad eating habits.

The attention should be shifted to being more disciplined towards your eating habits. Do not sit in front of plate stuffed with food items and eat in such a way, that you are forced to unbuckle the belt button while you finish it. Instead, enjoy eating smaller meals at regular interval, and that is healthy as well as tasty food. Along with it, you should spend an hour in regular exercise. Isn't it simple to follow? But the result will be fantastic as you will have higher control of your body. You won't ever become a slave of your cravings for food.

4. FIBER... ARE YOU GETTING ENOUGH?

How important is the role of fiber in our diet? Well, for your information, fiber is very helpful in fighting against certain common illness like diabetes, heart disease, diverticulitis and above all stroke. Moreover, it has an ability to control your desire for food. It gives you the feeling of contented with food; so that you will be able satisfy yourself with smaller quantity of food.

It is recommended to include at least 30 grams and 20 grams of fibre content in food for men and woman respectively. Fruits, vegetables, whole grain breads, etc are rich in fibre content. You can also try Raisin Bran Extra as a breakfast cereal as it includes 7 grams of fiber in it.

There is another point to consider regarding the intake of fibre. Suppose you eat 10-15 grams of fiber in a normal day. Make sure you do not suddenly switch to eating 30 grams a day. It is because the body needs time to adapt to a newer style. Slowly, you can replace low fiber foods with fiber-rich foods by giving time for your body to adapt to it.

We already discussed about milk shades in earlier chapters. There it was mentioned to prefer juice to milk shakes for its healthier content. A cup of apple or orange juice includes high amounts of fiber and low quantity of calories, which makes it a good choice of drink. Why don't you consider having a cup of juice along with the breakfast meal? Or even include grapes or bananas in your breakfast meal.

Crackers also makes a good option, when talking about fiber-rich food. For a great breakfast meal, whole wheat bread, crackers and cereals would make a great choice. Beans are another good source of fiber too. You can eat beans in your breakfast or lunch, as it also provides you with essential proteins.

5. HIT THE TREADMILL!

Exercise is not included in our routine life for many amongst us. It is often considered as an uphill task to get up early, and spend a few hours in exercise. It is pretty much easy to do nothing and weep over the obese body. To get the desired results of exercise, you need constant effort.

There are many options to include a little bit of physical exercise in your routine. You can use a machine like elliptical and chose not to run on the road. Why not use an exercise bike rather than biking down trails or rocky terrains? Don't you think it is quite easy to take your tennis racquet and play a game with your friends every evening? Tennis, boxing, bowling etc requires real physical movement and these are methods of enjoyment and strong physical activity. Incorporating any of this in your daily routine will surely do wonders on you.

Even if you have a problematic back or aching knees you can find a good exercise option that fits to you. It is not a reason to stay away from exercising. You can go for Wii Fit or similar gifts from the world of technology. It engages you in fun exercise routines and measures your fitness level and you realize the calories you burnt in the while.

If you are a person of 165 lbs, you are not going to lose 500 calories if you spend half an hour jogging or playing football or tennis. Instead, it takes time to get back in shape. Suppose you are new in the world of exercise, it will take lots more time to shed pounds. It is a method of engaging in healthier lifestyles by lesser intake of food and an hour of physical activity. You will get the desired results with time.

You can also divide up your exercise timings and continue it regularly. The best thing about cardio-type exercises is that you don't need to do it at a stretch. It can be done during different timings of the day and reach your goals. If you are in the habit of waking up at 6:30 am, try waking up thirty minutes before to engage in physical activity in a treadmill. It will refresh you and give a great start for the day.

Treadmill is never a must. You can go for a jogging session of 30 mts which will kill calories up to 500, depending on your fitness level. A brisk walk would also help you to burn about 200 calories. You can chose to go for a walk or jogging, or cycling, or engage in sports like soccer, basketball, tennis or whatever be your interest. The prime point is you need to sweat by engaging into a certain level of physical activity.

What to do in the winters or rainy season? Take a

membership in the nearest gym and get introduced to a number of cardio-machines like treadmill, exercise bike, elliptical, stair climber, rowing machine etc. Almost all machines are designed to get your heart pumping and will make you sweat. Be sure you start up slow and later get into fast practices. Give time for the body to adjust to the new regime and get the desired results over time.

6. WATER IS YOUR BEST FRIEND!

How much is the right amount of water you need? It is perhaps 8 glasses, if scientific research is taken into consideration. On a further note, it is actually calculated by dividing your weight by two. For example, if you weigh 180 lbs, divide it by two that equals 60. You can be sure you need 60 ounces of water a day.

Why is water important? It is considered essential for a healthy body and mind. It avoids dehydration. It promotes the proper functioning of your kidneys. It assists in the elimination of waste products from the body. It helps in the metabolism of the body. It also helps you to lose weight.

Experts will inform you more about the importance of drinking water. First and foremost, understand your body well. You will naturally drink water to quench your thirst. It is fine. But you have to monitor the type of work you do and be sure you drink more cups of water in accordance with the requirement. Keep a water bottle handy and make it a habit to drink water.

You have extra careful during hot summer days and hydrate your body with water intake at regular intervals. It is the time you sweat more and thus body loses water.

Life without water is simply impossible. To stay healthy and quench your thirst, you need water. You have to monitor the water intake and stay away from sugared drinks. Instead, drink water or juice or soda along with meals. It will reduce the calorie intake and gives you a better feeling.

.

CONCLUSION
READY... SET... GO!

People are well informed about many healthy dietary habits. They will go through numerous reading materials, and gain knowledge. The fact is only a few takes it into practical level. It is very difficult or impossible to lead a healthy life, unless you become disciplined and resist the temptation to have unhealthy foodstuffs. You need to motivate yourself to healthier food habits.

It is very easy to say "Yes, I can do it", but it needs effort to take the first step. You need to be really committed to get on the track of a healthy lifestyle. Many people will start with it and leave it in the middle since they need instant results.

If you want to achieve your goal, you need to be committed and self motivated. Let your goal be losing weight to becoming an athlete, you need to put strong effort.

Once you adjust to the training regime, you will be more disciplined. You will have a positive attitude and you will be more self confident. Thereby you can control the temptations.

It requires a start to achieve a goal anyway, let it be from anywhere. Break down your goals rather than desiring for instant results by setting up difficult goals. Start it slow, say by a brisk walk, and then slowly get into rigorous jogging in the following weeks.

People often start with rigorous exercise and it will be obviously painful and taxing. You can better start under a personal trainer and chose the one most comfortable for you, so that the process will be easy.

To conclude, all you need is to monitor the food intake and engage in physical activity to shed your pounds. Be confident and optimistic. Work towards your goals and you will get the desired results.

As we are approaching Spring, it is the time for a good beginning. Develop a plan for yourself and act on it to be on the road of a super healthy lifestyle.

Thank you and good luck!

WaraWaran Roongrungsri